Pathological demand avoidance explained

by Sally Cat

Foreword by Libby Hill

All royalties donated to PDA Socety

Foreword

Pathological Demand Avoidance (PDA) is such a difficult topic for most of us to understand yet Sally Cat's visuals, not only give us an insight into how the mind of a person with PDA works, she makes it appear logical. I always look forward to seeing her graphics so I was delighted to discover that she had presented them all in one place. Her designs are clever, quirky and compelling.

This is a great book to browse or to even to go through all in one go. It's perfect for showing people to explain more about the complexity that is PDA or, as I have used it already, to make a point. She includes everything we need to know from childhood through to adult life and everything in between. I have shown it to young children with PDA to help them understand themselves, siblings and family members. Ideal to present to teachers, professionals and employers.

Put it on your coffee table, you'll never be short of something to discuss.

Libby Hill, creator of SmallTalk Language Therapy who featured on C4's "Born Naughty!"

Contents

PDA stands for pathological demand avoidance.

It describes a neurotype (type of brain) which is classed as part of the autism spectrum.

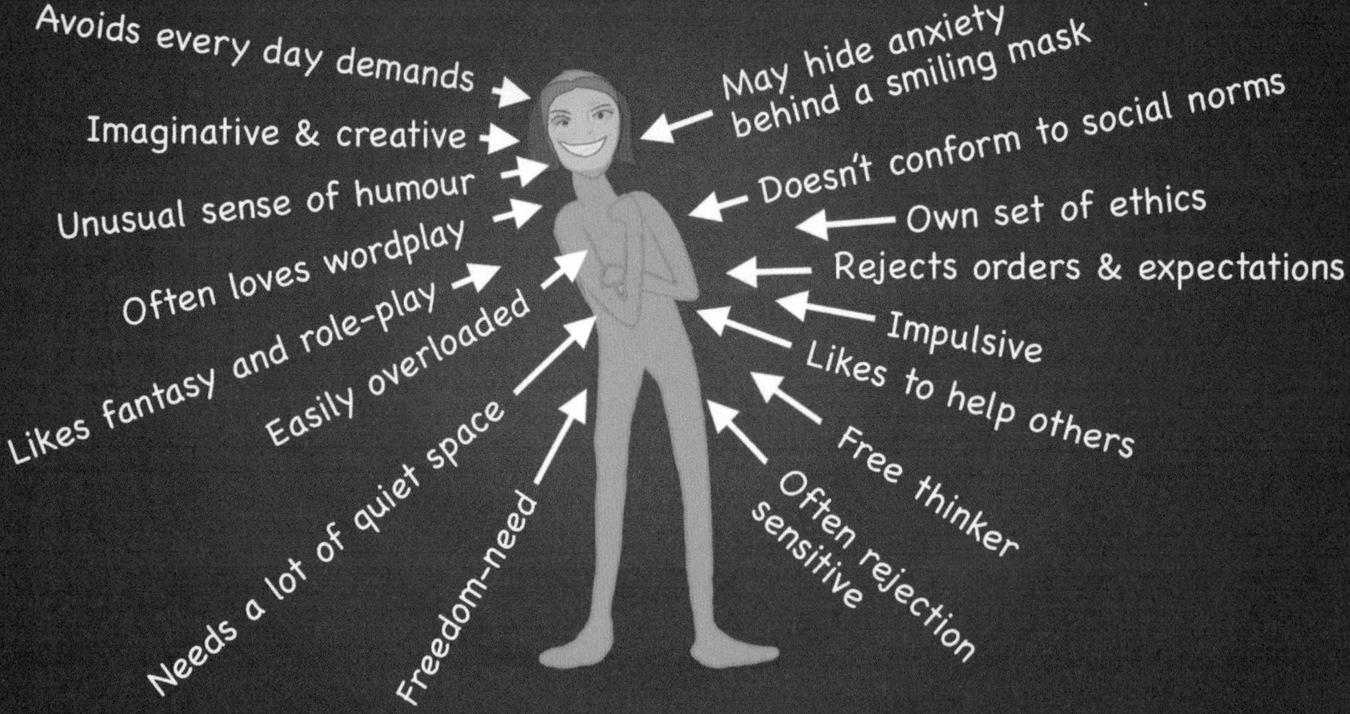

Part one: about PDA avoidance

GO ON!

I RECOMMEND

This section explores avoidance of the "pathological" kind:

How it works

What triggers it

What it feels like

2

How my PDA brain tells me I don't want things I had actually wanted

As soon as I think I want something, like a cake...

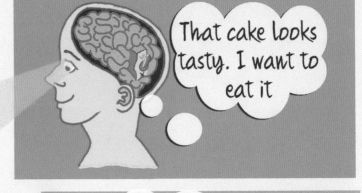

...my PDA avoidance clicks into action and tells me I don't want it after all

3

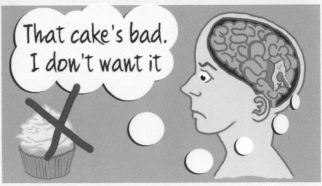

The PDA lens

My pathological demand avoidance acts like a distorting lens...

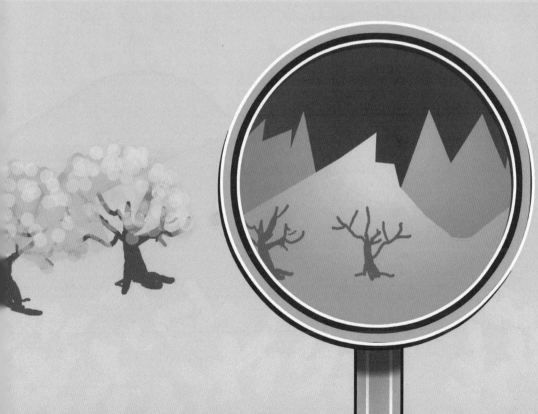

...Making pleasant things seem sinister so I want to avoid them

4

Set books at school

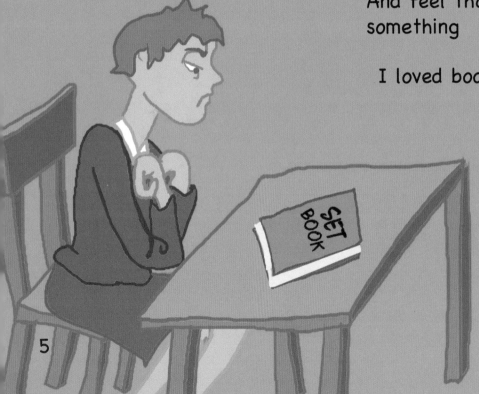

My PDA avoidance is triggered when I have no choice

And feel that I have to do something

I loved books as a child

But if a teacher set a book for us to read in school, that book felt like the most boring thing in the world

This was because I had no choice about reading it

Even gentle pressure

Like someone urging me with "please"

Feels like an attack

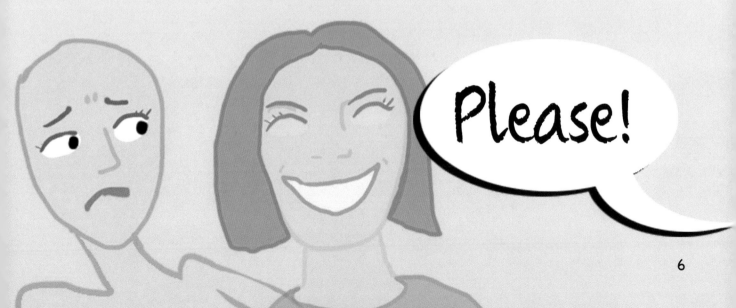

Please!

How different statements trigger my Demand Avoidance

STATEMENT	EXAMPLE	DEMAND AVOIDANCE
Command	You must go out	Ultra high
Aggressive command	Move it!	Ultra high
Pressuring	I'd like you to go out	Ultra high
Assumption	You'll love going here	High
Decisive suggestion	Let's go out!	High
Polite request	Please do come too	Medium/High
Unpressured suggestion	Maybe we could go out?	Medium/High
Unpushy opinion	I'd quite like to go out	Low
Consultation	Where's good for you?	Low
Unassuming	You're welcome to come	Low
Forbidding	You can't come	Inverted!

Inverted demand avoidance

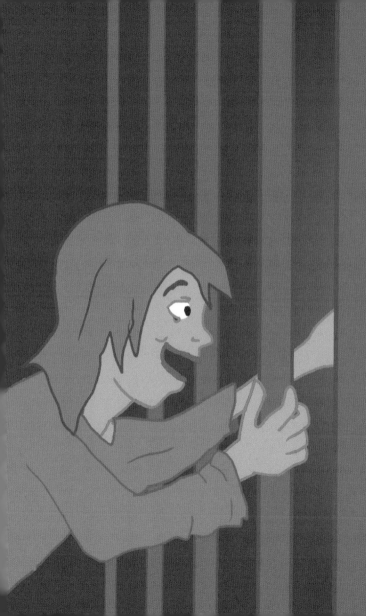

FORBIDDEN

If there's a demand for me not to have something...

...then I want it more than anything else in the world

The avoidance game

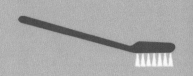

Demands can be anything and everything.

For example:

- Listening to music
- Reading a message
- Sticking to a schedule
- Brushing my teeth
- Eating fruit (which I actually enjoy)

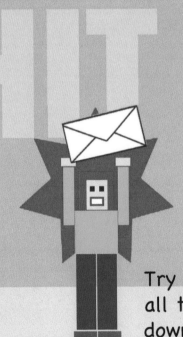

Try as I might, I can't avoid all the demands life hurls down on me

9

We PDAers can be creative in avoiding demands...

...sometimes using more energy in avoiding than it would take to actually do the thing!

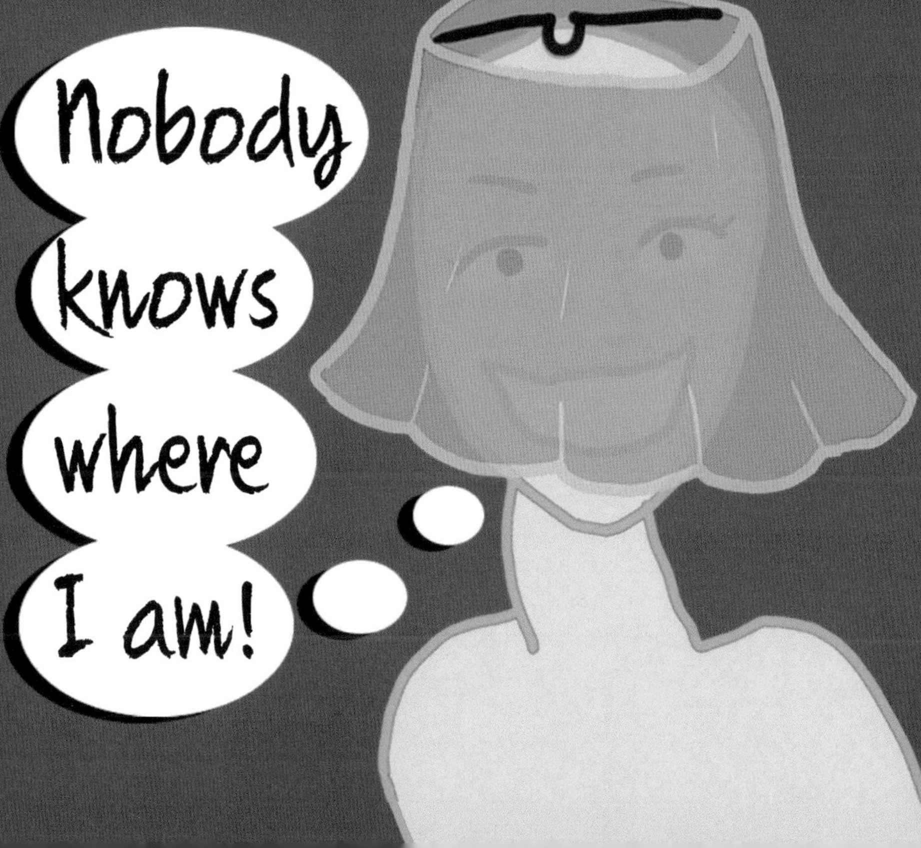

Feeling helpless

My PDA avoidance can make me feel helpless...

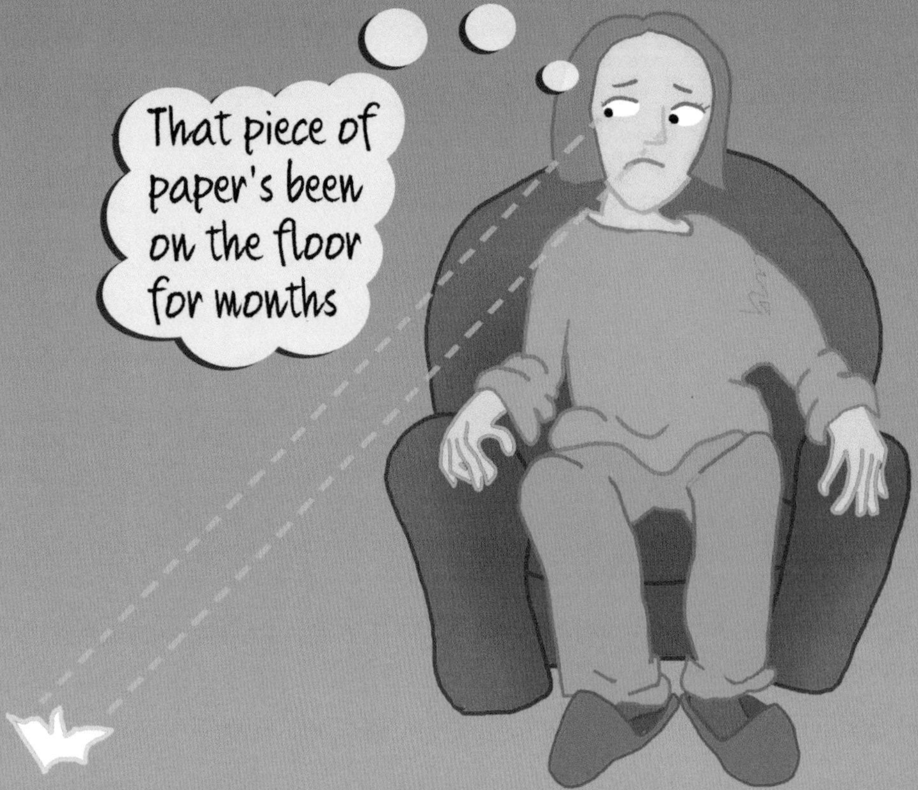

...so that even simple tasks, such as picking up a piece of paper from the floor, seem impossible...

...this can be confusing and frustrating!

When I was a child, if my mum told me I had to tidy my room,

And she wouldn't let me avoid it,

I'd sit there just looking at all the mess,

Feeling really anxious about it,

But unable to lift a finger to move
a single toy

12

Battling my demand avoidance can feel like trying to force two same-pole magnets together...

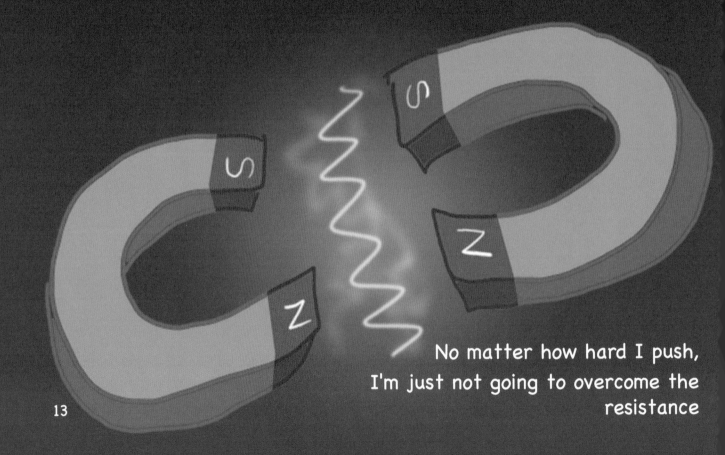

No matter how hard I push, I'm just not going to overcome the resistance

The emotional weight seesaw

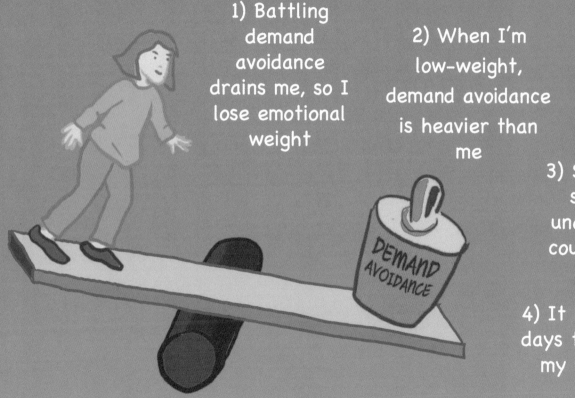

1) Battling demand avoidance drains me, so I lose emotional weight

2) When I'm low-weight, demand avoidance is heavier than me

3) So I am stuck unable to counter it

4) It can take days to regain my weight

DEMAND AVOIDANCE

I do not have the energy to meet all demands

Devil whispering on my shoulder

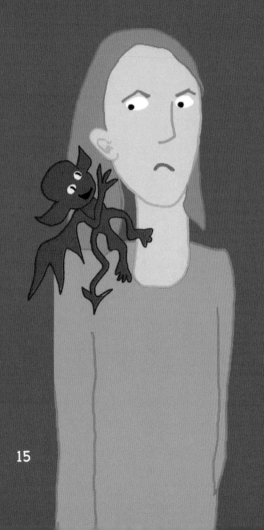

Every single thing I think to do is dampened by demand avoidance

This reaction has always been there

So I tend not to notice it

It runs in the background

Painlessly

(Pain only comes if I do not, or cannot avoid)

15

Invisible Demand Avoidance

Demand avoidance is not a loud response inside me

It is feather-light, and hard to feel

It's only really noticeable when I can't easily avoid things

Just like you only feel air when pressure makes it into wind.

My demand avoidance is not obvious unless demands are forced

Forcing triggers anxiety so my adrenaline fight / flight / freeze
response kicks in

Part two: about PDA control-need

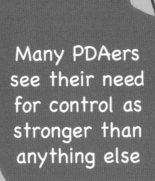

Many PDAers see their need for control as stronger than anything else

Understanding my control-need

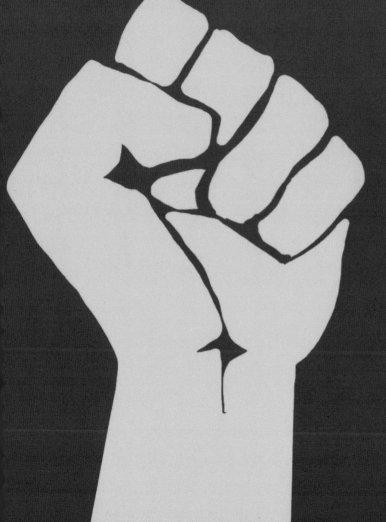

My need for control feels like part of my demand avoidance

When I am in control, there are no external demands on me

(Although I may still be plagued by niggly internal ones, like pieces of paper I think I should pick up)

18

Anxiety from control-loss

Lack of control causes me high anxiety...

...because it means I can't avoid demands

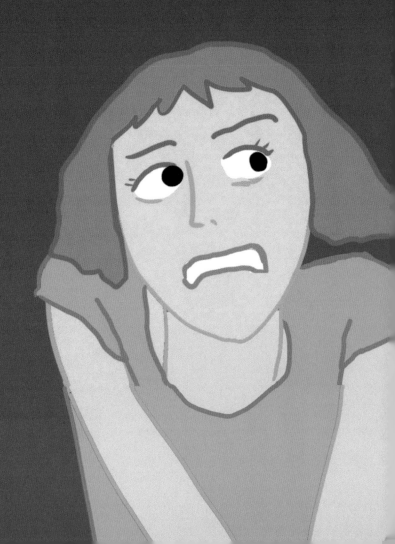

A poem about my contrariness

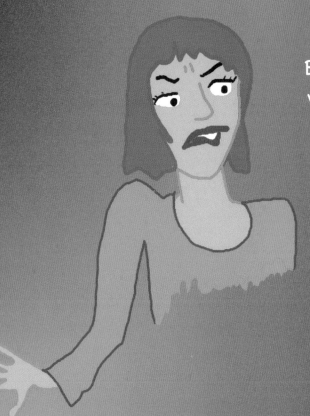

I need control of my life,
And struggle to be free,
But control spills onto others,
When I only meant 'just me'.

And I'm hurt beyond
endurance
When criticised by you,
But I criticise lik crazy
The things that others do

Personal Control

I denied I wanted to be in control
for much of my life because I didn't
want to be a bad "control freak"

I now understand that
my need is to be in
control of my own life
(not of others).

I think our PDA need
for control shapes us
to be free thinkers.

Freedom Need

I think control is a way of
maintaining FREEDOM

(Which my PDA causes me to need)

So I think my
demand
avoidance is
caused by my
desperate and
natural need to
be free

If people try to control me

No matter how
politely,

And regardless
of their place
in social
hierarchy,

It feels like they
are attacking me.

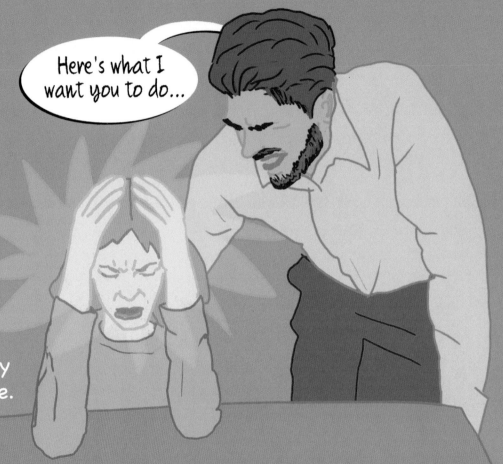

23

Part three: about PDA anxiety

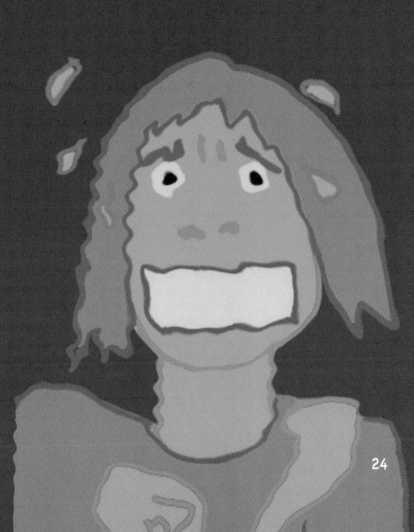

PDA involves having very high anxiety...

...but we may not always be aware of it

24

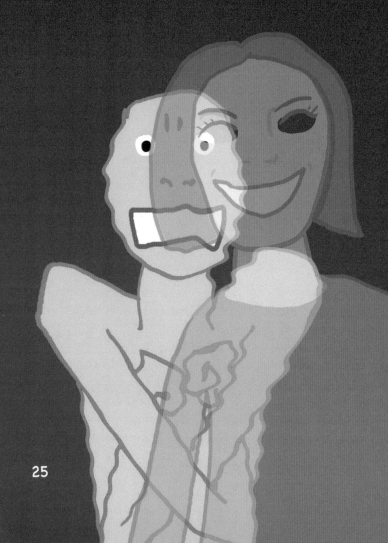

Natural PDA anxiety

We are born
with it

It's not
something
that comes from having had
bad experiences (although
these can make it worse)

My high anxiety was so
normal that I didn't notice
it for much of my life.

25

Anxiety-Blindness

I've realised I had so much constant anxiety that it was my normal state

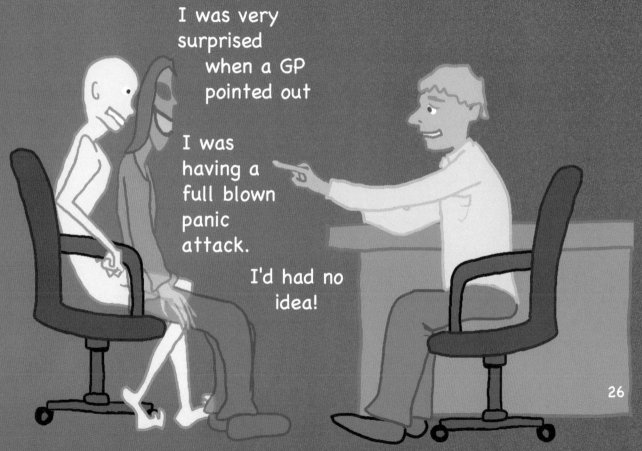

I was very surprised when a GP pointed out

I was having a full blown panic attack.

I'd had no idea!

ANXIOUS THOUGHTS

that person's watching me, I don't like it

that big task still needs doing

my house is a mess, but I don't want to have to clean it

I've got visitors coming round next month

everyone hates me

did I embarrass myself?

I don't want to make that phone call

I might be seriously ill

I spent all the money again

I don't know what I'm supposed to say

I should bathe, but I don't want to

The Fear-Wall

I've always
had a wall of
fear that springs
up around me when I
think about doing
certain things, or if I
try to speak to people
I don't know well

I've never wanted the
fear-wall there...

...or known how to
make it go away

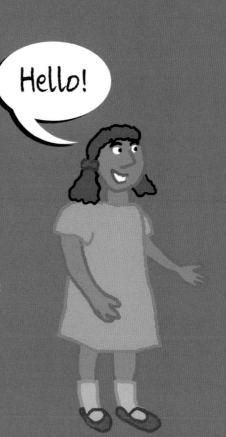

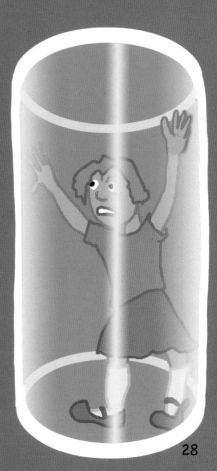

28

Social Anxiety

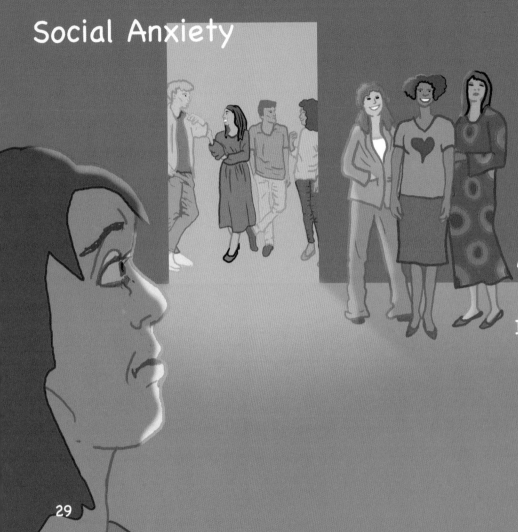

I want to join in,

But I don't feel worthy.

There's something wrong with me.

I can't just let go,

And laugh and have fun.

I can't relax and be natural like everyone else.

I wish I could.

I really do.

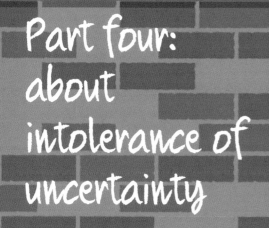

Part four: about intolerance of uncertainty

A study carried out by Newcastle University found that intolerance of is even higher for PDA children than anxiety...

30

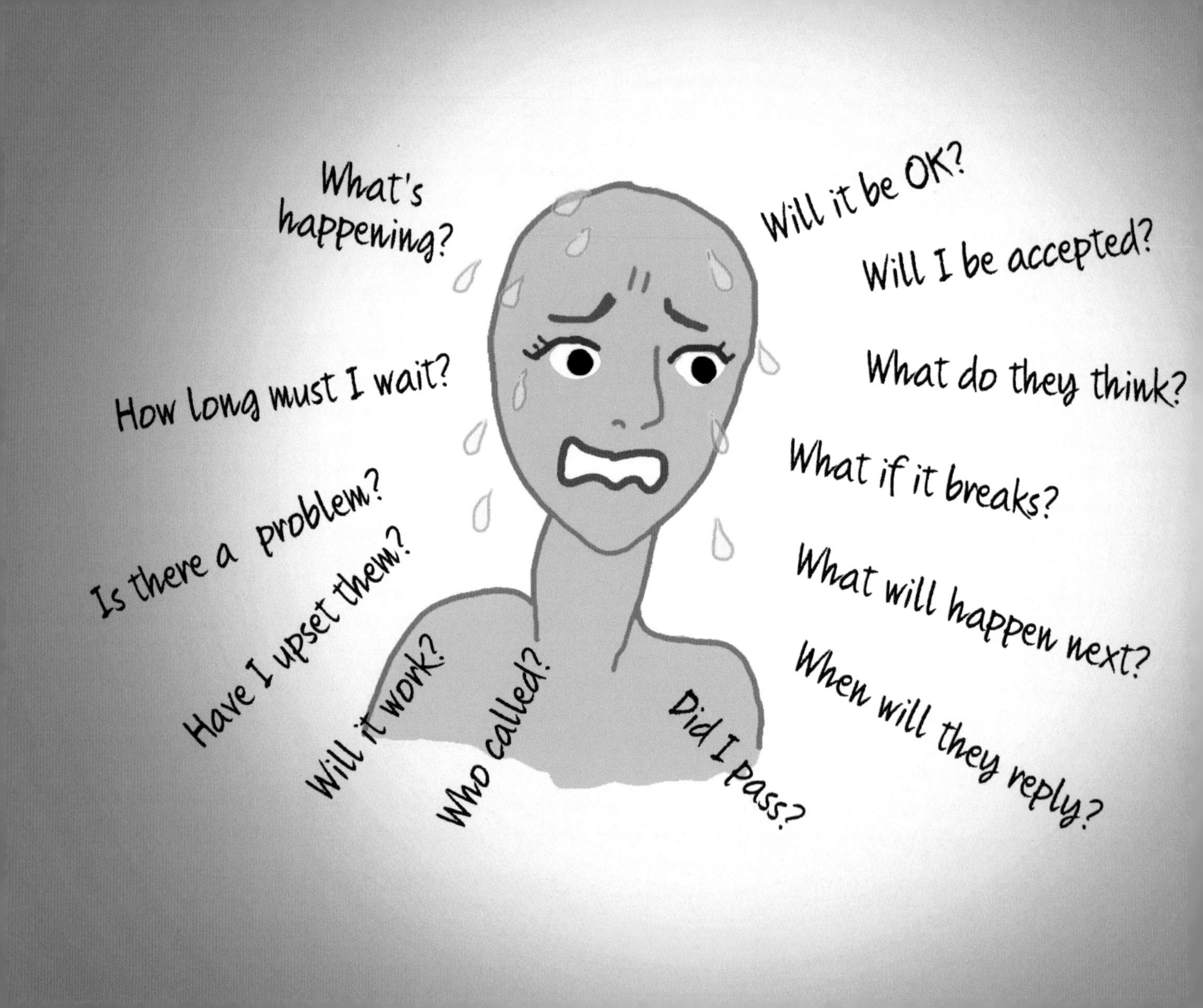
What's happening?
Will it be OK?
Will I be accepted?
How long must I wait?
What do they think?
What if it breaks?
Is there a problem?
Have I upset them?
What will happen next?
Will it work?
Who called?
Did I pass?
When will they reply?

Childhood intolerance of uncertainty & TV

What's going on?

As a child, I was desperate to know what was happening in TV shows I watched with my family

I sensed that my constant questioning was annoying to my parents

But my need to know was greater than my desire not to be annoying!

Intolerance of uncertainty when kept waiting

I find it intolerably stressful if I'm kept waiting, say for a doctor's appointment, for longer than twenty minutes...

Factor in stresses from the demand of having to stay there; bright lights; the noise of people talking, etc...

...and I am very likely to overload and march out before being seen!

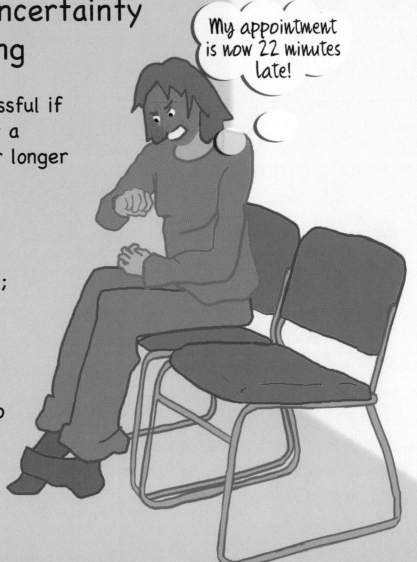

Part five: about PDA social mimicry & masking*

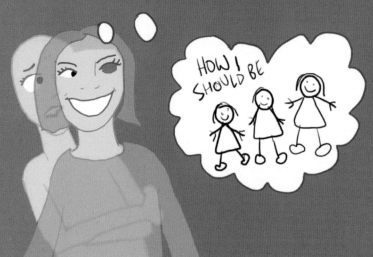

HOW I SHOULD BE

Masking = hiding your true feelings, often by putting on a calm or happy expression

Social mimicry = copying what you think is the right behaviour to fit in with other people

* Some PDAers say they don't mask at all

34

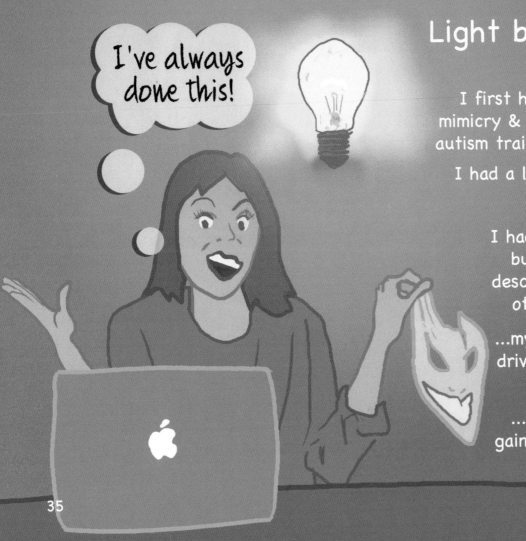

Light bulb moment

I first heard about social mimicry & masking in a female autism traits list I found online

I had a light bulb moment:

I had always done this, but never heard it described as something other people did...

...my lifelong masking-drive started to make sense...

...and I sought and gained an adult autism diagnosis

Are general autistic & PDA masking different?

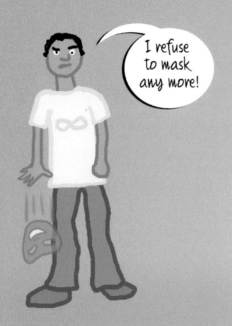

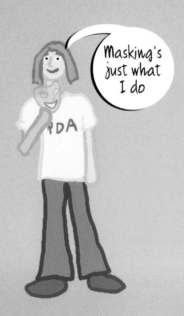

Autistic people tend to see masking as an evil thing forced on them by society

And view it as an unhealthy habit they can give up

PDAers seem more likely to see masking as natural

And that we couldn't give it up, even if we tried

36

How masking helps me talk to people

I find it hard to speak to
people because of my
fear wall, and not
knowing what to say

I build masks from things
I've learned people react
well to

Knowing I can say and do the
right thing pokes a hole
through my fear-wall

So I'm able to talk to people
and sometimes make friends

It's important to me to be able to do this

Constructing tailor-made masks

I build special masks for
people I value in my life

I have to shape them just
right to match each person

This takes a lot of time
and effort

But once it's fine-tuned, I
can talk to that special
person almost effortlessly

I think this is why I tend to
have just one or two close
friends at a time

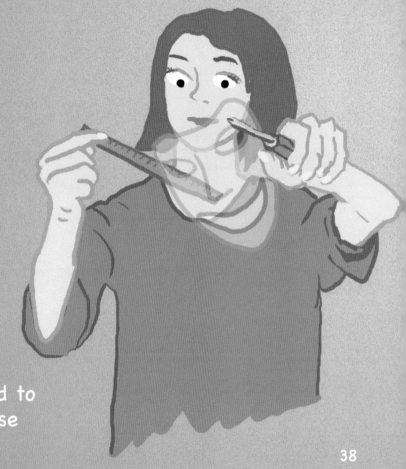

38

Turning on charm

I can use my mask to be charming to people

I use eye contact, even though I find it uncomfortable

I do this to let people know they're special to me

And to come across as interested and engaged

Part six: about PDA emotions

Having strong, rapidly changing emotions (including anxiety) is a recognised trait of PDA

40

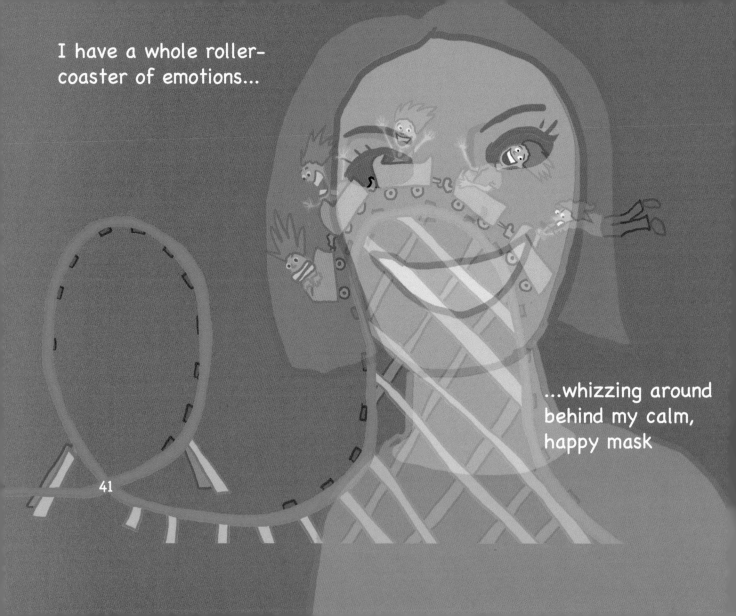

Emotion blindness (alexythemia)

I've always struggled to recognise & name my emotions
But this doesn't mean I've not felt anything,
I've always felt loads.

I don't know what I feel

What's all this havoc in my head?

Why do I keep finding situations really hard to cope with?

What is anger? I don't think I feel it

Why did I just shout at them?

I just feel... I don't know what, but I'm finding life incredibly difficult now

What's wrong with me?

42

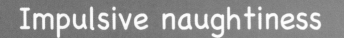

Impulsive naughtiness

I sometimes feel compelled to do naughty things...

That's so funny!

...just because they're funny...

...even if other people don't think they're funny at all...

...these impulses always involve breaking demands of how I'm expected to behave

POO

43

Compulsive attachments

As a child & younger adult,
I often found myself obsessed
by certain people or groups
who seemed glamorous

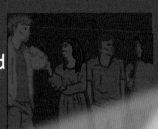

My desire for them could
be totally overwhelming

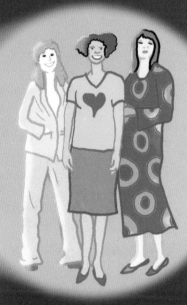

Those people are so
cool. I must have
them in my life!

It would take over my
thoughts, and drive me mad

44

Rejection sensitive dysphoria (RSD)

RSD is extreme, overwhelming emotional pain when I feel rejected

It feels like sharp knives stabbing into my body and cutting it open

I can't think about anything else,
No matter how hard I try

It can take months, even years to recover

(Although RSD is thought of as an ADHD thing, many PDAers, say they experience it too)

45

Fierce protector-mode

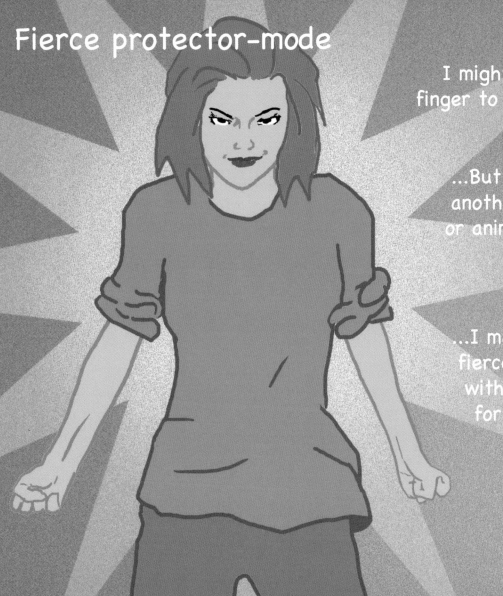

I might not lift a finger to help myself...

...But if I come across another person, group, or animal being treated unfairly...

...I may launch into my fierce protector mode without any thought for my own safety

Part seven: about PDA overload, meltdown & shutdown

Overload = brain strained from too much pressure

Meltdown = brain-processing explodes like a bomb

Shutdown = brain switches off & stops working

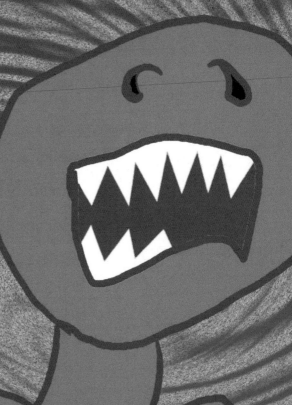

About overload

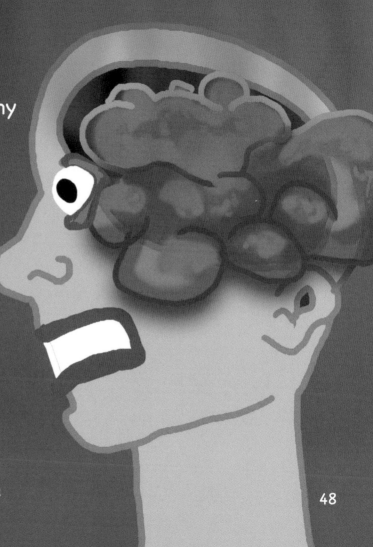

I become overloaded if there is more stuff coming at me than my brain can cope with

Some of the things that can overload me are:

> Bright light
>
> People talking
>
> Demands I can't avoid
>
> Being kept waiting

My brain feels hot, painful and squashed

I can't cope with anything else

48

Overload and people

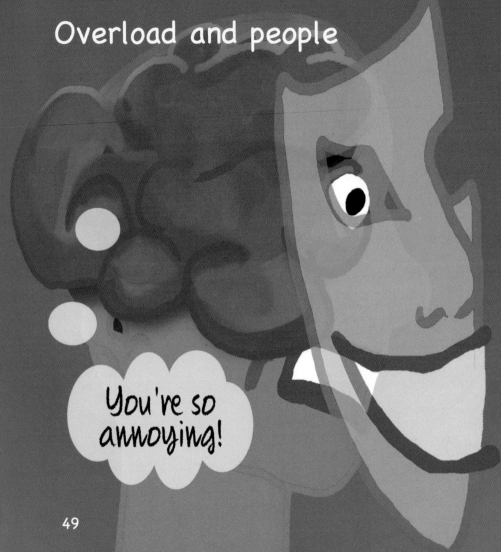

I find it very hard to keep up my calm, friendly mask when I'm overloaded

Even though I want to

My overloaded brain cannot take any more.

I feel:
 Irritible
 Impatient
 Attacked
 Unable to think clea

I have often fallen out with people wh
like this

49

How overload causes meltdown & shutdown

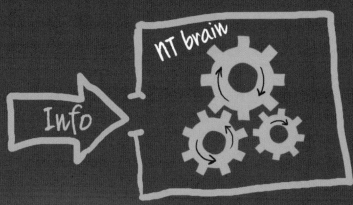

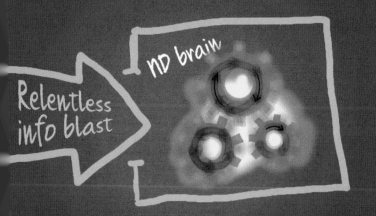

1) If you think of typical brains as machines efficiently filtering & processing incoming information...

2) ...neurodiverse brains have less filter, so they get bombarded and overload quickly,

Unless they have many breaks from input in which to catch up with processing

3) Without breaks, the machine will either meltdown or shutdown

50

Me excited thinking about having quiet time soon

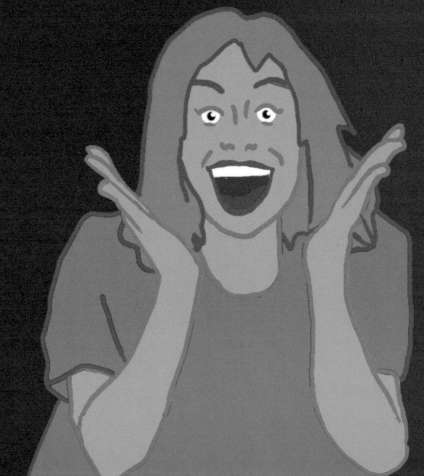

Quiet time need

For me quiet time is not a luxury to fit in only if there's spare time,

But a top priority.

If I don't have quiet time...

...and a lot of it...

...I go into meltdown or shutdown

52

Screen time

I spend a lot of time messing around on
my phone

I used to feel guilty for this,

I thought it was unhealthy &
lazy

But now I know I need this
idle screen time to
recharge my brain

And avoid overload

Resisting quiet time

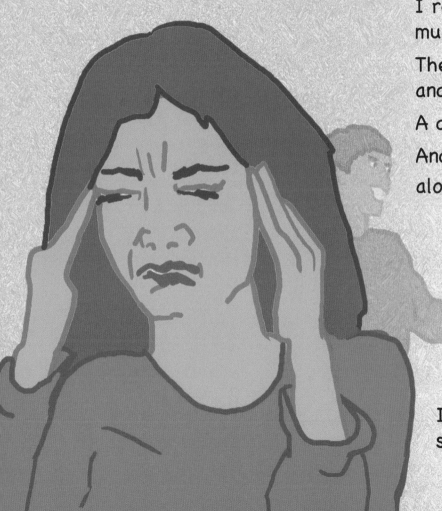

I resisted quiet time for much of my life.

The idea of it felt bleak and boring;

A demand to do nothing,

And the thought of being alone was scary

I used to get very, very stressed!!

54

Meltdown is not a choice

Meltdown happens if I overload

No amount of discipline makes it stop

When I meltdown, I have no control over my words & actions

My best strategy is to avoid overload so meltdown doesn't happen to begin with

Trying to control myself during a meltdown...

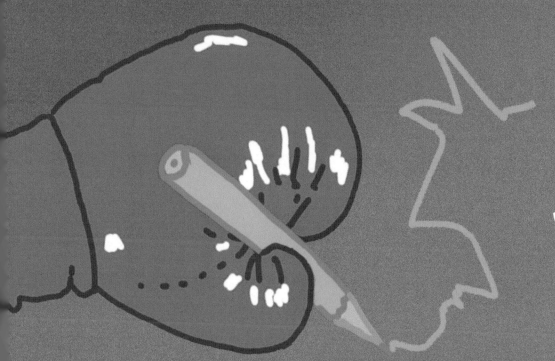

...is like trying to draw a neat line while wearing a boxing glove

56

Feeling like I'm possessed

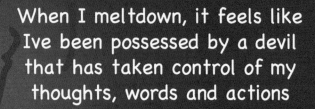

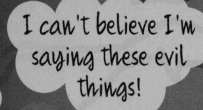

I can't believe I'm saying these evil things!

When I meltdown, it feels like Ive been possessed by a devil that has taken control of my thoughts, words and actions

This devil uses my memories & knowledge to hurt those around me

While I watch on in helpless horror,

Feeling shocked & ashamed at myself for saying & doing such terrible, spiteful things

57

What is shutdown?

Shutdown, like meltdown,
is something that
happens when my brain
overloads

My brain stops working,
like a machine with stuck
cogs

My thoughts won't start,

My words are gone,

My body can't even

Unlike meltdown, shutdown is a
very quiet reaction

58

Recovering from meltdown & shutdown

As for avoiding them in the first place, recovering from meltdown and shutdown requires lots of quiet time so my brain can cool down & start working again

MELTDOWN

SHUTDOWN

QUIET TIME

59

Part eight: about PDA & school

70% of parents reported that their PDA children were either not enrolled in a school, or struggling 'all the time' or 'regularly' to get in.

(PDA Society 2018)

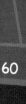

Help me!

I was like a fish out of water at school

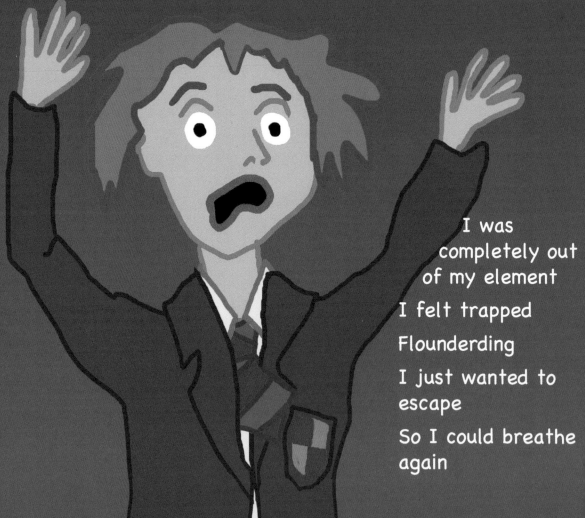

I was completely out of my element

I felt trapped

Flounderding

I just wanted to escape

So I could breathe again

Demands in school

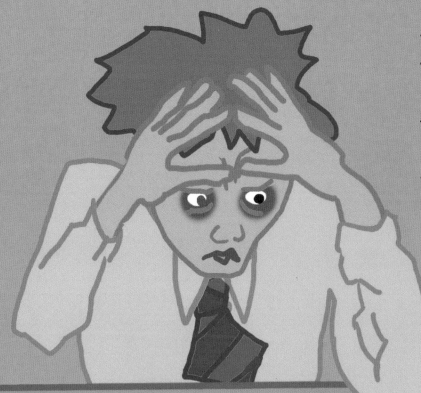

School was a battlefield of demands.
I had to crush myself to comply:

Turn up every school day
Wear uniform
Sit at your desk
Do as you're told
Learn what we command
Behave as we say
  Do not leave until we
  allow it
Have no control
Do not be free

Or find a way
to escape...

Can't wake early

My demand avoidance & anxiety about going to school was made worse by a condition called "delayed sleep phase syndrome"

I've had this since I was a young child

It means my body's clock is set to much later than other people's...

...so no matter how tired I've been in the day, I can never get to sleep until very late at night... Waking up as early as most people means I've not had enough sleep

63

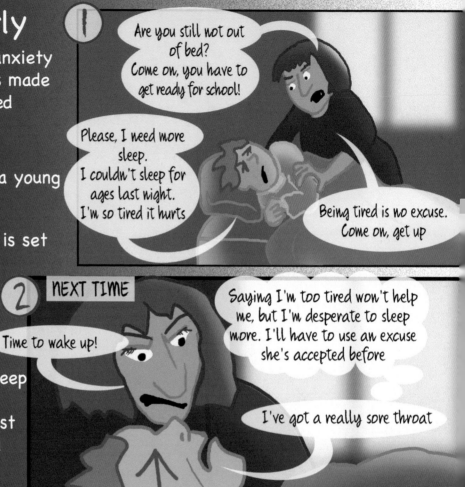

School art block

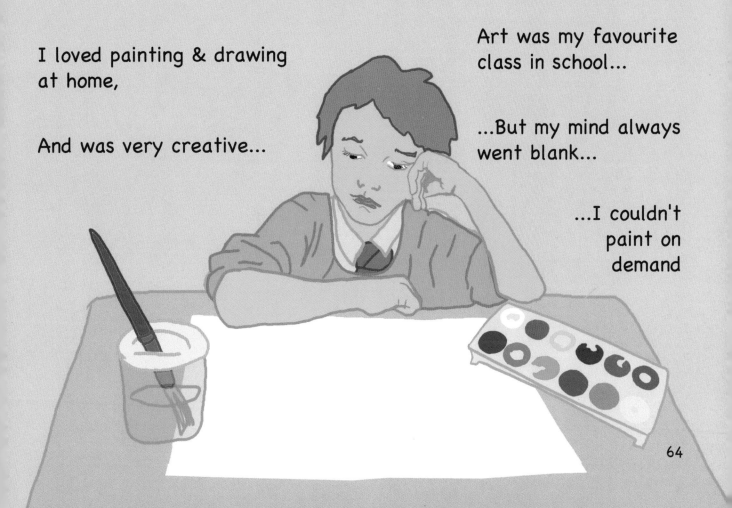

I loved painting & drawing at home,

And was very creative...

Art was my favourite class in school...

...But my mind always went blank...

...I couldn't paint on demand

Alone in the playground

I had trouble making friends at school

I didn't know why, but the other children didn't want to play with me

I didn't know why, but the other children didn't want to play with me

I got on OK with the boys until I was seven...

...then, when school started again after the summer holiday...

...the boys didn't want to play with me either

I felt sad, alone, confused & certain that there was something very wrong with me

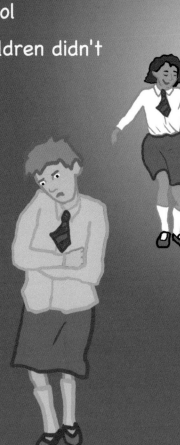

Happy daydreams

Daydreaming gave me some
happiness at school

The stories I daydreamed
were very complicated

I was always the hero...

...popular, strong and in control...

...I preferred my daydream stories to
reality

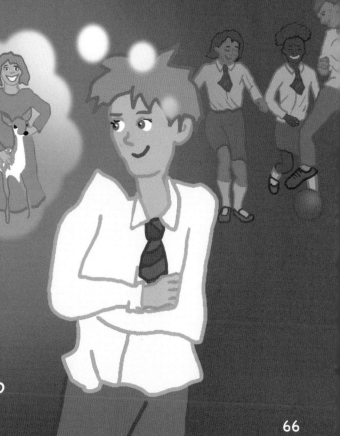

66

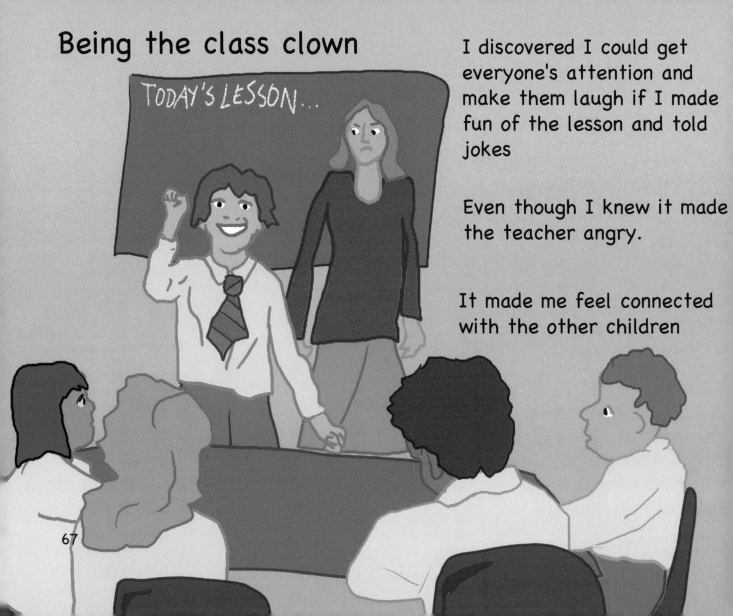

Skipping school

I escaped school as much as I could

Because I hated it

It felt like a punishing prison sentence

I used all my imagination to find ways to avoid it

Pretending to be ill didn't always work...

...so I took to telling my parents I was going to school, and wandering the streets...

...and giving my teacher forged sick notes when I finally returned

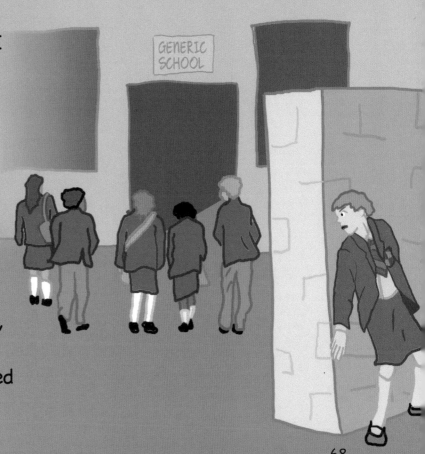

The happiest moment of my life

Finishing school for ever
was the happiest moment
of my life...

...but all the
other girls were
crying...

...I never
wanted to seem
like an alien...

...so I
pretended
to be sad
and tearful
too

69

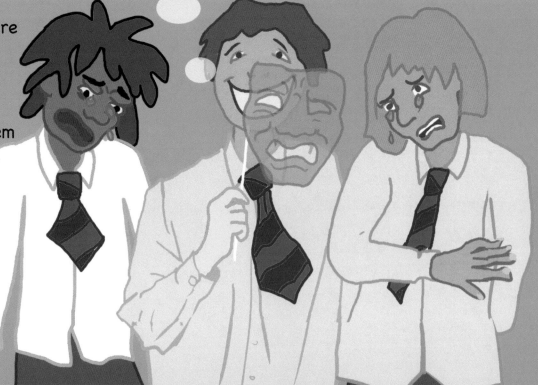

Part nine: adult life

Being an adult has never come easily to me!

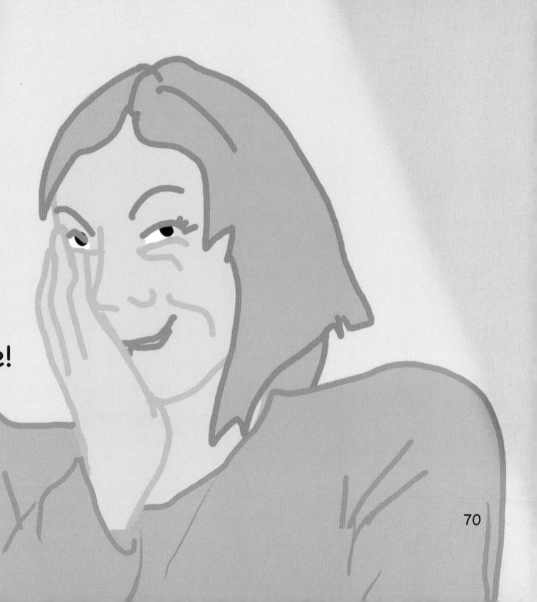

Career choices

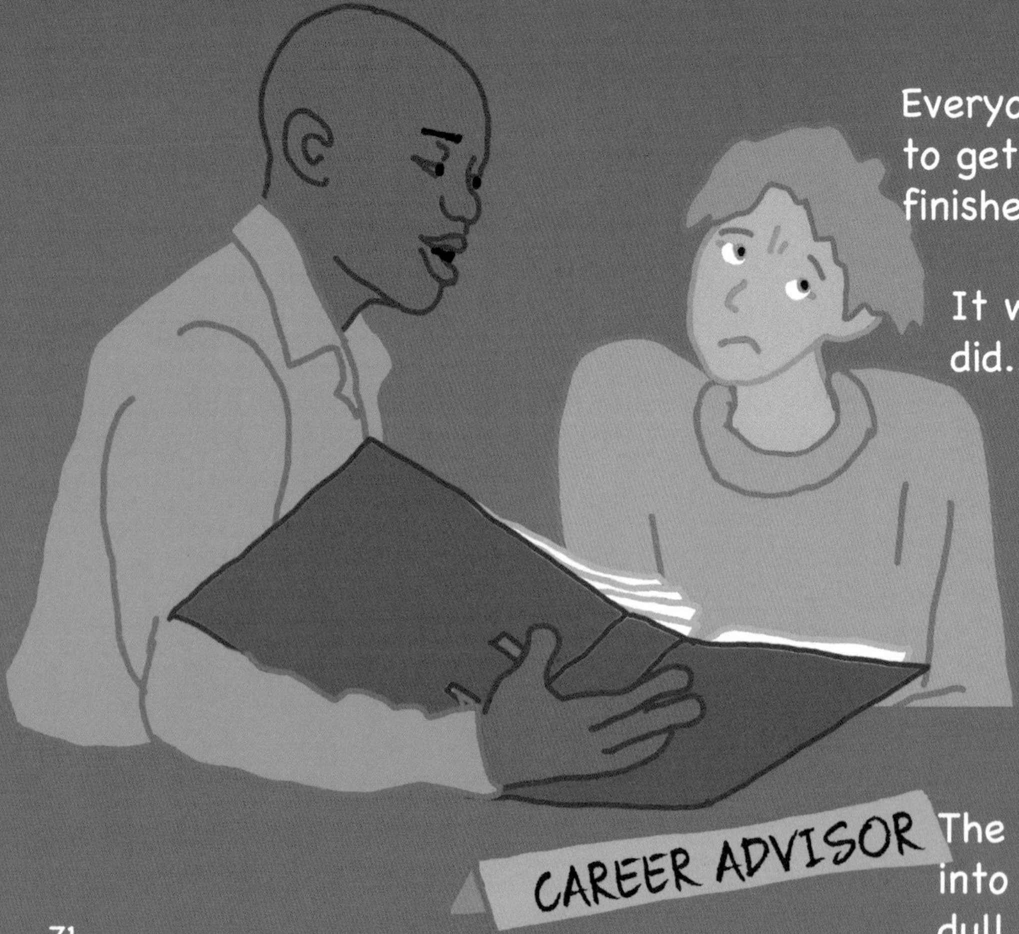

Everyone expected me to get a job when I finished school

It was what everyone did...

...so I thought I should want one.

But of all possible career ideas,

Not a single one was appealing

The idea of entering into them felt like dull versions of Hell!

Fleeing jobs

Every time I've tried working to earn a wage

I've felt trapped very quickly,

And miserable and stressed until I've got away.

The more I've got used to a job,
the more unbearable it felt

So it was never long until I fled

How long till I can leave?!

SERVICE

72

Career-less

I've never been able to stay in jobs long
enough to earn a livable wage

I was rubbish at budgeting what little
money I did have

I couldn't afford enough food

I got into trouble with the police

I did dangerous things

And felt totally alienated from society

I liked to get drunk to forget my failures,
And social anxiety

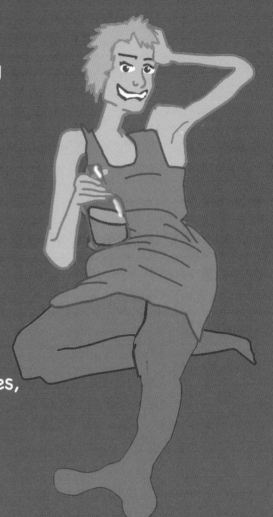

73

Demand avoidance triggered by pay

I have flourished in many voluntary roles

Where I've had creative freedom

I love to feel useful and helpful

But the moment someone offers to pay me

No matter how desperate I am for money

I feel enslaved

I lose all motivation and inspiration

And just want to be free of it

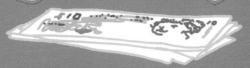

74

The positive power of neurotype awareness

I spent most of my adult life chronically depressed,

Because, unlike those around me, I couldn't get into a career, and earn money to live on.

I ran up debt

And struggled to eat & pay bills

Discovering PDA, and how it impacts me was an uplifting revelation

I no longer feel depressed about what I can't do, and am achieving the most I ever have

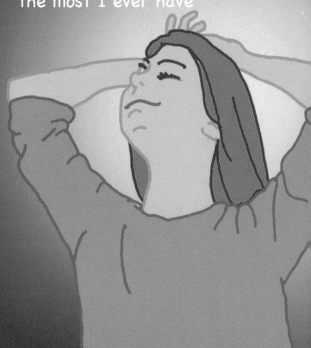

If you have found my memes helpful, you can see many more of them on my Facebook page: facebook.com/SallyCatPDA/

I also have a blog: sallycatpda.co.uk

Write for Free PDA: www.freepda.co.uk

And authored the first book about adult PDA, "PDA by PDAers" which was published by JKP in 2018

But no demand ever ;)

Sally Cat

Printed in Great Britain
by Amazon